NUTRITION AND WELLNESS: A COMPREHENSIVE GUIDE FOR NEWBORN AND BREASTFEEDING MOTHERS

EMPOWERING MOTHERS:

ESSENTIAL NUTRITION FOR THE FIRST STEPS OF LIFE, NOURISHING YOUR BABY THE RIGHT WAY, A DETAILED GUIDE TO MATERNAL NUTRITION AND INFANT HEALTH.

NANCY SPEARS

TABLE OF CONTENT

INTRODUCTION

Importance of nutrition for newborns and breastfeeding mothers

Breast milk is the ideal meal for newborns and infants. A nursing woman's nutritional resources may be depleted to some extent as a result of pregnancy and blood loss after childbirth. Lactation increases nutritional requirements, primarily due to nutrient loss from colostrum and breast milk.

Breastmilk amount varies greatly. The nutrients in this milk are derived from the mother's food or nutritional reserves.

Nutrient conversion from meals to breast milk is incomplete. To maintain optimal nutritional status, the breastfeeding mother must increase nutrient intake. Human breastmilk has a relatively consistent composition and is only selectively changed by the mother's diet. The fat content of breastmilk varies slightly. Even if the mother's diet lacks certain nutrients, the carbohydrate, protein, fat, calcium, and iron contents remain rather stable. A mother whose diet is weak in thiamine, as well as vitamins A and D, produces less of these nutrients in her milk. The mother should be instructed to follow a varied diet. At each postnatal appointment, both the mother and the baby should be evaluated, and advice on both mothers' and infants' nutrition should be given. The easiest approach to determine the sufficiency of an infant's nutrition is to see if he or she gains enough weight. Mothers should not get less than 1800 calories each day.

During breastfeeding, a mother must pay attention to the nutrients that enter her body. Nutrition for breastfeeding women not only promotes physical health but also the production of breast milk, which is essential for the baby's growth and development.

Breastfeeding women can meet their nutritional needs in a variety of ways, including taking supplements and eating healthful meals. The provision of essential nutrients is critical not only for the mother's health but also for the development of the child. So, what nutrients are required by breastfeeding mothers?

Breast milk must provide adequate nutrition for the newborn as a continuation of intrauterine nutrition, and both the mother's nutritional state and food may influence breast milk composition, and hence nutrient intake in the infant.

Nutritional requirements are higher in infancy than at any other stage of development, and there is evidence that the content of breast milk changes throughout time to meet the changing needs of the child.

Although there is a wealth of information on the physiology and pathology of lactating mothers, the professionals who care for them frequently lack knowledge of their nutritional needs. This paper seeks to provide up-to-date information on breastfeeding mother nutrition to aid in the formulation of current knowledge-based healthcare procedures.

Women's nutritional requirements rise during pregnancy and nursing. During breastfeeding, the mammary glands have a certain level of metabolic autonomy that ensures proper milk composition. Unless they are very malnourished, all moms are capable of producing adequate volumes and quality milk.

Variations in the mother's diet may cause changes in the fatty acid profile and levels of certain micronutrients, but they are not related to the volume or quality of milk produced. All mothers' milk, even if malnourished, is of outstanding nutritional and immunological quality. The mother's body constantly prioritizes the baby's needs, thus most nutrients including iron, zinc, folate, calcium, and copper continue to be excreted in breast milk in adequate and consistent amounts, at the expense of maternal storage. In the event of famines and disasters, particularly when there is a risk of infant malnutrition, the WHO recommends supporting breastfeeding to ensure the baby's proper growth, as well as supplementing the mother's diet.

Human milk contains energy, proteins, and nutrients derived from both the diet and maternal body storage. Women who do not get enough nutrients from their diets may be deficient in certain minerals and vitamins that are essential for their health. These deficiencies can be avoided if the mother alters her diet or takes nutritional supplements.

Age, baseline postpartum weight, level of exercise, and individual metabolism all determine how much food each woman needs to consume to achieve optimal nutritional status and an adequate milk supply. The duration and intensity of breastfeeding have a major impact on mothers' nutritional needs, yet they are rarely taken into account.

The frequency of nutritional deficiencies varies by geographic region, culture, dietary habits, and socioeconomic status. In Spain, micronutrient shortages are more prevalent than calorie or protein deficiencies. Some nutrients in human milk are determined by the mother's food intake, particularly if her diet is poor, and these shortages may usually be rectified with supplements.

The amount of water-soluble vitamins in breast milk is greatly reliant on mother consumption. Fat-soluble vitamin concentrations are primarily dependent on maternal reserves, but they can be boosted by exogenous sources.

It has been proven that maternal needs vary depending on the stage of lactation. Women can avoid shortages throughout pregnancy and lactation by getting enough energy and eating a balanced diet that includes fruits, vegetables, and animal-sourced meals. Some nutrient requirements, particularly those for iron, iodine, folic acid, and vitamin A, are more difficult to meet from dietary sources, therefore women may need to take supplements or eat fortified foods.

CHAPTER ONE

Understanding Nutrition for Newborns and Breastfeeding Mothers

Get to know breast milk basics

A nutritious diet is crucial not just for maintaining your overall well-being but also for ensuring that your kid receives all the necessary nutrients to flourish.

Except for vitamin D, breast milk contains everything your baby needs for normal development throughout the first 6 months.

Insufficient nutrient intake in your overall diet can have a negative impact on both the quality of your breast milk and your health.

Breast milk consists of 87% water, 7% carbohydrate, 3.8% fat, and 1% protein and delivers 65–75 calories per 100-milliliter amount.

Unlike baby formula, breast milk varies in calorie quantity and composition. The composition of your breast milk undergoes dynamic changes at each feeding and throughout your lactation period to cater to the specific requirements of your infant.

At the beginning of a feeding, the milk is more watery and usually quenches your baby's thirst. The subsequent milk, known as hindmilk, is denser, richer in fat, and more nourishing.

This milk may include 2–3 times as much fat as milk at the beginning of a feeding and 7–11 more calories per ounce.

Hence, to obtain the most nourishing milk, it is necessary for your infant to fully drain one breast before transitioning to the other.

Enhance your consumption of foods that are rich in nutrients.

The act of nursing can significantly increase your appetite levels, leading to a notable increase in hunger. The process of producing breast milk places significant physiological demands on the body, necessitating an increased intake of calories and bigger quantities of particular nutrients.

Health professionals approximate that the energy requirements during nursing rise by around 500 calories per day.

Your needs for the following essential nutrients also increase:

• protein

• vitamin D

• vitamin A

• vitamin E

• vitamin C

• vitamin B12

• selenium

• zinc

This is why eating a range of nutrient-dense, whole foods is so vital for your health and your baby's health. Choosing meals rich in the above nutrients can help guarantee that you obtain all the macro- and micronutrients you and your little one need.

Here are some nutritious and enjoyable food choices you might seek to prioritize during breastfeeding:

• Fish and seafood: salmon, seaweed, shellfish, sardines

• Meat and poultry: chicken, beef, lamb, pork, organ meats (such as liver)

• Fruits and vegetables: berries, tomatoes, bell peppers, cabbage, kale, garlic, broccoli

• Nuts and seeds: almonds, walnuts, chia seeds, hemp seeds, flaxseed

• Healthy fats: avocados, olive oil, coconut, eggs, full-fat yogurt

• Fiber-rich starches: potatoes, butternut squash, sweet potatoes, beans, lentils, oats, quinoa, buckwheat

• Other foods: tofu, dark chocolate, kimchi, sauerkraut

But you're not confined to these foods. Check out this list for more ideas for nutrient-dense ingredients.

Also, while enjoying your favorite foods on occasion is healthy, it's important to decrease your intake of highly processed foods such as fast food and sugary breakfast cereals as much as possible.

For example, if you're used to starting your day with a huge bowl of brightly colored breakfast cereal, you may try substituting it with a bowl of oats topped with berries, unsweetened coconut, and a dab of nut butter for a satisfying and healthy fuel source.

Adjust your breastfeeding diet for both nutrient groups

The nutrients in breast milk can be divided into two classes, based on the extent to which they are released into your milk.

If you're deficient in any group 1 nutrients, they won't secrete into your breast milk as quickly. Supplementing these nutrients can give a tiny boost to their concentration in your breast milk and benefit your baby's health as a result.

On the other hand, the concentration of group 2 nutrients in breast milk does not depend on how much you take in, thus supplementing won't improve your breast milk's nutrient concentration. Even so, these nutrients can boost your health by replenishing your nutrient storage.

If all of that seems a little confusing, no worries. Here's the bottom line: Getting enough group 1 nutrients is crucial for both you and your baby, whereas getting enough group 2 nutrients is primarily only necessary for you.

Group 1 nutrients

Here are the group 1 nutrients and some frequent food sources of each one:

• Vitamin B1 (thiamine): fish, pork, seeds, almonds, beans

• Vitamin B2 (riboflavin): cheese, almonds, pecans, red meat, fatty seafood, eggs

• Vitamin B6: chickpeas, nuts, salmon, chicken, potatoes, bananas, dried fruit

• Vitamin B12: shellfish, liver, yogurt, oily fish, nutritious yeast, eggs, crab, shrimp

• Choline: eggs, cow liver, chicken liver, fish, peanuts

• Vitamin A: sweet potatoes, carrots, dark leafy greens, organ meats, eggs

• Vitamin D: cod liver oil, oily seafood, certain mushrooms, fortified foods

• Selenium: Brazil nuts, shellfish, turkey, whole wheat, seeds

• Iodine: dried seaweed, cod, milk, iodized salt

Group 2 nutrients

Here are the group 2 nutrients and some typical food sources:

• Folate: beans, lentils, leafy greens, asparagus, avocados

• Calcium: milk, yogurt, cheese, leafy greens, legumes

• Iron: red meat, pig, poultry, seafood, beans, green vegetables, dried fruit

- Copper: shellfish, whole grains, nuts, beans, organ meats, potatoes

- Zinc: oysters, red meat, poultry, beans, almonds, dairy

The concentration of group 2 nutrients in your breast milk is relatively unchanged by your dietary intake and your body's storage of those nutrients.

So, if your intake is low, your body will extract these nutrients from your bone and tissue stores to secrete them into your breast milk.

Your kid will always get the appropriate amount, but your body's stores will deplete if you don't ingest enough. To avoid deficiencies, you need to receive enough of these nutrients from your food or supplementation.

Consider taking supplements

Although a balanced diet is the most important component in nutrition when nursing, no question that taking supplements can assist in replenishing your stocks of certain vitamins and minerals.

There are various reasons you can be low in key nutrients during the postpartum period. You might not be eating enough of the foods that provide those nutrients or meeting the increased energy requirement of breast milk production. Plus, your diet may have changed while you're busy looking after your newborn.

Taking supplements can help enhance your intake of critical nutrients. However, it's vital to be vigilant when choosing supplements since many contain herbs and other ingredients that aren't healthy for breastfeeding parents.

We've put up a list of nutrients that are beneficial for breastfeeding parents and for improving postpartum recovery in general. Always be sure to purchase products from reputed manufacturers that undergo testing by third-party organizations such as NSF and USP.

Multivitamins

A multivitamin can be an excellent method to enhance your consumption of key vitamins and minerals.

Vitamin and mineral shortages are frequent after delivery, and research reveals that deficits affect birthing people in both high-income and low-income settings.

For this reason, it may be a good idea to take a daily multivitamin, especially if you don't think you're getting enough vitamins and minerals through your food alone.

Vitamin B12

Vitamin B12 is an extremely vital water-soluble vitamin that's essential for your baby's well-being and your health during nursing.

Plus, many people — especially those who follow largely plant-based diets, have undergone gastric bypass surgery, or take certain medications (such as acid reflux meds) — are already at an elevated risk of having low B12 levels.

If you belong to one of these groups, or if you believe that you don't get enough B12-rich foods (such as fish, meat, poultry, eggs, and fortified foods), then taking a B-complex or B12 supplement is a smart option.

Remember that most high-quality multivitamins and prenatal supplements contain enough B12 to satisfy your needs.

Omega-3 DHA

Omega-3 fatty acids are all the rage nowadays, and for good reason. These fats, naturally abundant in fatty fish and algae, play crucial functions in both your and your baby's health.

For example, the omega-3 lipid docosahexaenoic acid (DHA) is crucial for developing your baby's nervous system, skin, and eyes. And the concentration of this essential fat in breast milk mostly depends on your dietary levels.

Babies that ingest breast milk with high levels of DHA have superior vision and neurodevelopment results.

Because the amounts of omega-3s in your breast milk mirror your diet of these vital fats, you must eat enough. We propose that breastfeeding parents take 250–375 mg per day of DHA and eicosapentaenoic acid (EPA), another key omega-3 fat.

Although eating 8–12 ounces of fish — especially fatty fish like salmon and sardines — will help you reach the required dietary levels, taking a fish oil or krill oil supplement is a handy approach to cover your daily needs.

Vitamin D

Vitamin D is found in only a few foods, such as fatty fish, fish liver oils, and fortified goods. Your body can also create it with sunshine exposure, though your vitamin D production relies on numerous factors, such as your skin color and where you reside.

This vitamin serves numerous key roles in your body and is essential for immune function and bone health.

Vitamin D is normally available in relatively modest amounts in breast milk, especially when sun exposure is limited.

Supplementing 400 international units (IU) of vitamin D per day is advised for breastfed newborns and babies eating less than 1 liter of formula per day, commencing in the first few days of birth and continuing until 12 months of age.

Supplementing with 6,400 IU per day can help supply your infant with enough amounts of vitamin D through breast milk alone. Interestingly, this amount is substantially greater than the current recommended vitamin D consumption of 600 IU for breastfeeding parents.

Vitamin D insufficiency is especially common among people who are breastfeeding. Deficiency can lead to unfavorable health effects, including an increased risk of postpartum depression. That's why supplementing with this vitamin is recommended.

Ask your healthcare provider for exact dose recommendations based on your current vitamin D levels.

Drink plenty of water

In addition to being hungrier than usual while breastfeeding, you may feel thirstier.

When your infant latches onto your breast, your oxytocin levels increase, causing your milk to start flowing. This also promotes thirst and helps ensure that you stay hydrated when feeding your baby.

Your hydration needs will vary depending on factors such as your exercise levels and nutritional intake. There's no one-size-fits-all suggestion for how much hydration you need during breastfeeding.

As a general guideline, you should always drink when you're thirsty and until you've quenched your thirst.

But if you feel particularly fatigued or weak or fear your milk production is dropping, you may need to drink extra water. The simplest way to tell whether you're drinking enough water is to pay attention to the color and smell of your urine.

If it's dark yellow and has a strong smell, that's a sign that you're dehydrated and need to drink more water.

Foods and drinks to restrict or avoid when breastfeeding

Although you may have heard differently, it's fine to consume just about any food while breastfeeding unless you have an allergy to a specific item.

While some flavors from food, spices, or beverages may influence the taste of your breast milk, research shows that those changes are unlikely to affect your baby's feeding time or make them irritable.

Another prevalent misunderstanding is that "gassy" foods like cauliflower and cabbage may promote gassiness in your infant too. Although some foods may make you gassy, the gas-promoting chemicals do not transfer to breast milk.

In summary, most foods and drinks are acceptable during nursing, but there are a handful that are best to limit or avoid. If you think something may be badly harming your kid, consult your healthcare expert for advice.

Caffeine

About 1% of the caffeine you consume is passed to breast milk, and newborns take significantly longer to metabolize caffeine than adults do. Drinking caffeinated beverages such as coffee has not been found to cause harm but may impair your baby's sleep.

Therefore, health experts recommend reducing your coffee intake to 2–3 cups per day while you're breastfeeding. It's a disappointment, we know, but at least some coffee is allowed, right?

Alcohol

Alcohol can also make its way into breast milk. The concentration resembles the amount present in the breastfeeding parent's blood. But babies metabolize alcohol at only half the rate that adults do.

Nursing after drinking only 1–2 drinks might lower your baby's milk intake by up to 23% and cause anxiety and poor sleep.

Because drinking alcohol too close to breastfeeding might severely affect your baby's health you should limit your alcohol intake while you're breastfeeding.

It is recommended to ingest no more than 0.5 grams of alcohol per kilogram of body weight. For a 60-kilogram (132-pound) individual, that is 2 ounces of liquor, 8 ounces of wine, or 2 beers.

While it's normal to enjoy an alcoholic beverage as a breastfeeding parent, it's preferable to wait at least 2 hours after drinking to nurse your infant.

Cow's milk

Although it's unusual, some babies are allergic to cow's milk. If your kid has a cow's milk allergy, you must remove all dairy items from your diet.

Up to 1% of breastfed newborns have an allergy to cow's milk protein from the breastfeeding parent's diet and may develop rashes, dermatitis, diarrhea, bloody stools, vomiting, or colic.

Your healthcare expert can advise you on how long to avoid dairy from your diet and when it's acceptable to reintroduce dairy.

Breastfeeding and weight loss

You might be tempted to lose weight rapidly after delivery, but weight reduction takes time, and it's crucial to be fair to your body throughout this transition.

As a result of the many hormonal changes that take place during breastfeeding and the calorie demands of making breast milk, you may have a bigger appetite during breastfeeding.

Restricting your calorie intake too much, especially during the first few months of nursing, may lower your milk production and much-needed energy levels.

Breastfeeding alone has been to promote weight loss, especially when continued for 6 months or longer. However, weight loss during breastfeeding doesn't happen for everyone.

Losing about 1.1 pounds (0.5 kilograms) per week through a combination of a healthy diet and exercise should not affect your milk supply or milk composition, assuming that you're not undernourished to begin with.

All breastfeeding parents, no matter their weight, should consume enough calories. But if your body weight is low, you'll likely be more sensitive to calorie restriction.

For this reason, if you have a low body weight, it's essential to consume more calories to avoid a reduction in milk supply.

All in all, remember that losing weight after delivery is a marathon, not a sprint. It took months to put on the weight for a healthy pregnancy for both you and your baby, and it may take you months to lose it — and that's OK.

The most important thing to remember when trying to lose pregnancy weight is that restrictive diets are not good for overall health and don't work for long-term weight loss.

Following a nutritious diet, adding exercise into your daily routine, and getting enough sleep are the best ways to promote healthy weight loss.

CHAPTER TWO

Preparing Your Kitchen

Essential kitchen tools for preparing baby food

Cooking baby meals is pretty simple! All you need to do is make sure the food is soft (at the start) and either purée or mash it. The equipment you need to prep, cook, mash, and purée isn't that complicated. Most are probably already in your kitchen.

Prep

Peeler

A sharp peeler speeds up the process of peeling your fruits and veggies. Most purées (at least at the start) are produced without skin for uniformity and digestive ease. Apples, squash, carrots, potatoes... you'll need to peel, so pick a nice one!

Knives.

Every kitchen needs one decent chopping knife and a nice cutting board.

Cook Pots and steamer.

Pots and a metal strainer or some form of food steamer. I had the Baby Miter All in One and it was fantastic. I could steam/cook and combine in one shot. An InstantPot would have been amazing at that time too! But, all early purées start here. If you already have a variety of pots, you may just acquire a steamer to insert inside. Steamer inserts are handy so you may steam more than one batch of fruits or veggies at a time.

Baking sheets.

Baked food provides a whole new level to your baby's experience, therefore a large one is good to have ready.

Mini muffin tin. This is an excellent pan for creating little amounts. You'll need small paper liners for lining the cups.

Food thermometer.

Skip it if your family doesn't consume meat, but I believe this to be crucial for evaluating whether meat is done.

Blending

Blender or food processor.

This is going to be your best friend. Whether it's purées, smoothies, or soups, your blender or food processor will get a ton of use. Invest in a nice one so it lasts a long time, you'll know it was worth it when it's still working for five years. The better items on the market are quite potent, which can decrease your prep time in half. I have been using mine for 2 years and know I will be for as long as I'm cooking healthy meals, especially when you want to sneak some veggies in muffins or pancakes. ☐

Freeze and thaw

Silicone storage trays.

This might be just ice cube trays, or you can find the molds for baby food alone. Worth it to get the quantities down and store them in the freezer. Just make sure whatever you choose has a cover to guard against freezer burn.

Small glass bottles and jars.

These are ideal for thawing your frozen cubes of goodness. Many of them fit well in a bottle warmer!

Store

Small glass lockable containers or mason jars. I have a set of baby food containers, glass with seals and locking lids. The greatest best thing ever! I still use them for lunches. They are the perfect size.

Labeling

Frozen pea purées and green bean purées don't look all that different from one another. You'll want stickers and a marker if you make a lot and freeze. Especially when you start combining items and have options for breakfast or dinner.

Serving Spoons

Early on, I recommend a soft silicone-based spoon. As kids become older and those teeth come in, a firmer spoon with a deeper bowl is best.

Bowls

Part of the success of those first bites is getting your infant comfortable with the experience of eating. This indicates sitting down to a meal. Make yours and baby's plates together and sit down so mealtime becomes routine and family bonding time.

CHAPTER 3

RECIPES FOR BREASTFEEDING MOTHERS

Recipe 1: Quinoa and Vegetable Stir-fry

Key ingredients

Don't fret about the lengthy-looking ingredient list---it's mostly veggies and you don't have to use them all. The peanut sauce couldn't be easier to make.

Did I mention it's a dream drizzled on veggies and all the things?

- Quinoa: The base of our stir fry! Packed with protein, nutty-tasting, and quick-cooking. It's technically a seed (that's what they mean by "pseudo-grain.") I used white quinoa for this recipe, but you could also use red or tri-color.

- Veggies: Bell pepper, carrot, broccoli, and bok choy are my go-to for this meal but you can use whatever veggies, fresh or frozen, you have on hand.

- Aromatics: Plenty of onion, garlic, and ginger for flavor!

- Peanut butter: This makes the sauce super creamy and crave-worthy. I love Costco's organic creamy peanut butter in the sauce, but whatever peanut butter you fancy will do. Or even almond butter!

- Soy sauce: The best salty, umami flavor to form our yummy sauce.

- Maple syrup: A bit of natural sweetness helps round out all the flavors.

- Sesame oil: I love sesame oil in Asian-inspired dishes! Olive oil works, too.

- Lime: A bit of bright acidity for balance.

- Sriracha: I love a tiny bit of heat. Red pepper flakes work too!

How to cook quinoa

1. Rinse quinoa under cold water with a fine mesh strainer to get rid of the bitter-tasting outer layer.

2. Place in a small saucepan with 1 ¼ cups water. (I typically do a ratio of 1 part quinoa to 1 ½ parts liquid).

3. Bring to a boil over high heat. Once boiling, reduce heat to low and cover. Simmer for about 15 minutes, or until the liquid has absorbed and quinoa looks fluffy.

4. Fluff with a fork, transfer to a medium bowl and allow it to cool.

Time-saving tips

- Use pre-cooked quinoa if you so please! Or rice! It's a thing. You can find it in the frozen section of most grocery stores. Time is money, people.

- Try frozen veggies. I get massive bags of frozen stir-fry veggies at Costco that I often use in place of fresh veggies so I don't have to chop anything. It saves tons of time!

- Use fridge leftovers! This stir fry is forgiving. Peppers, mushrooms, cabbage, green beans, zucchini, asparagus, wild greens...throw them in the mix. The more veggies the merrier.

Go dried. Use garlic powder, bottled ginger (or dried!), and bottled lime juice (I always have this one on hand) if you don't have fresh. No shame!

Health benefits of quinoa
 quinoa because it's a complete plant protein with all 9 essential amino acids, trumping the protein content of other whole grains.

It's also higher in minerals like calcium, magnesium, iron, copper, and zinc (compared to corn, rice, and wheat). It has a good amount of filling fiber as well.

Why do you rinse quinoa?
Quinoa has naturally occurring compounds called saponins that taste bitter. They need to be rinsed off for optimal flavor! Some come pre-rinsed so check the package.

Simply rinse quinoa in a fine mesh sieve until it's no longer foamy then proceed with cooking.

How to store

Store leftovers in an air-tight container in the fridge. They will keep for up to three days. Reheat it in the microwave or a pan on the stove.

Can you freeze stir fry?

Yes! You can freeze it for up to 3 months.

Instructions

1. Place quinoa and water in a medium pot with 3 cups of water. Bring to a boil then reduce heat to low and simmer, covered, for 15 minutes. Fluff with a fork and set aside.

2. Meanwhile, whisk together the sauce ingredients in a medium bowl and set aside.

3. Heat olive oil in a **Dutch oven** or large pot over medium heat. Once hot, add onion, peppers, carrots, and a pinch of salt. Cook for about 7 minutes, or until softened. Add garlic, ginger, and broccoli, cooking for another 5 minutes or until broccoli is softened. Stir in edamame and bok choy at the end, cooking just until wilted.

4. Add cooked quinoa and sauce to the veggie mixture, stirring to combine. Taste and adjust seasoning as needed. Serve warm garnished with green onions and sesame seeds.

Recipe 2: Lentil Soup

Is lentil soup good for you?

If you're wondering if lentil soup is good for you, the answer is *yes!* Lentils are nutritious, rich in minerals, and protein, low in fat, and high in fibre (digestive health). They are a terrific vegetarian source of protein with 25% of the calories in lentils attributable to protein.

Lentils are a carbohydrate, but it's slow burning which means it keeps you fuller for longer. Studies also suggest that lentils are good for heart health.

The added benefit is that they are low in calories with 116 calories in 1 cup of cooked lentils (which is roughly the amount per serving of this lentil soup).

What does lentil soup taste like?

It tastes savory and has a flavor boost from a hint of spices. There's an undertone of natural sweetness from the *soffrito* flavor base of onion, carrot, and celery. My favorite part is the texture! It's thick and comforting, and just made for dunking in hot crusty bread!

What goes in Lentil Soup

Here's what goes in my lentil soup. Nothing fancy, just everyday ingredients.

So what makes this Lentil Soup so good?

- A touch of spices.

- Cooking the onion, carrot, and celery slowly so they sweeten and make a beautiful flavor base.

- Lemon – The "secret" ingredient. Yes really. A little tip I picked up from Ina Garten. Just a bit of zest and a squeeze of fresh lemon makes all the difference which takes it from really good to great!

Do you cook lentils before adding them to soup?

Nope! Dried lentils cook for 35 minutes *in* the soup, and there's no need to soak them either!

What type of lentils are best for lentil soup?

Dried lentils are best for lentil soup. You can use most types of lentils for this recipe – brown, green, red, or yellow, though it will affect the color of the soup. I've used green lentils, pictured below.

The only type of lentil I do not recommend is Puy Lentils (little black French lentils) because they hold their shape and don't soften like other lentils.

Can you use canned cooked lentils?

Yes, you sure can, and directions are provided in the recipe notes. But it's better made with dried lentils because of the texture in the soup, there's only a 10-minute difference in cooking time and it's more economical!

How to make Lentil Soup from scratch

- Sauté your onion, garlic, carrots, and celery over low heat for almost 10 minutes. Take your time here – the lower the heat, the longer you take, and the more these will transform to create an incredible flavor base for the soup!

- Add everything else other than the lemon;

- Simmer for 35 minutes until lentils are soft; and

- Finish with a dusting of zest and a spritz of lemon.

A hint of lemon earthiness from the zest and a touch of freshness from the juice just jazzes up the soup and takes it to that next level!

You'll find that the lentils mostly break down and naturally thicken the soup. But what I like to do to get a luscious creamy texture is to give the soup a quick whizz with a blender stick (or transfer a couple of cups to the blender) to puree SOME but not all the lentils.

That way you get the benefit of both worlds – creamy soup with soft bits of lentils. YES!

How to store lentil soup

Lentil Soup will easily be kept for 5 days in the fridge, making it ideal for cooking on the weekend and serving throughout the week. And it also freezes 100% perfectly for 3 months – even longer!

Every time I make this, I always wonder why I don't make it more often. It's healthy, filling, super economical, freezes perfectly, versatile and it's seriously good.

Serving this with some sort of warm crusty bread for dunking is not optional. It's an essential part of the Lentil Soup experience.

But it is optional whether you slather said bread with butter, or grill it with cheese! Here are a few options – including making your ultra-easy **homemade bread with NO YEAST**:

Ingredients

- ➢ 2 tbsp olive oil
- ➢ 1 onion, chopped *(white, brown, yellow)*
- ➢ 2 garlic cloves, minced
- ➢ 1 large carrot, *chopped (about 1 1/4 cups)*
- ➢ 2 celery ribs, *chopped (about 1 1/4 cups)*

➢ 2 cups / 400g dried lentils, *green or brown, rinsed (Note 1)*
➢ 400g / 14 oz crushed tomato
➢ 1.5 liters / 1.5 quarts (6 cups) vegetable or chicken *stock/broth, low sodium*
➢ 1/2 tsp each cumin and coriander powder
➢ 1 1/2 tsp paprika powder
➢ 2 dried bay leaves
➢ 1 lemon (zest + juice)
➢ 1/4 tsp salt and pepper, *each*

Instructions

1. Heat oil in a large pot over medium heat. Add garlic and onion, and cook for 2 minutes.

2. Add celery and carrots. Cook for 7 - 10 minutes or until softened and the onion is sweet. Don't rush this step, it is key to the flavor base of the soup.

3. Add all remaining ingredients except the lemon and salt. Stir.

4. Increase heat and bring to a simmer. Scoop scum on the surface off and discard (do this again during cooking if required). Place the lid on and turn the heat down to medium-low. Simmer for 35 - 40 minutes or until

lentils are soft.

5. Remove bay leaves.

6. Thicken Soup: Using a stick blender, do 2 or 3 quick whizzes to thicken the soup (see video below). Or transfer 2 cups to a blender, let it cool slightly, then hold the lid with a tea towel and blend then transfer back into the pot.

7. Add a touch of water if you want to adjust soup consistency. Season to taste with salt and pepper. Grate over the zest of the lemon then add a squeeze of lemon juice just before serving. Garnish with parsley if desired and serve with warm crusty bread slathered liberally with butter!

Recipe Notes:

1. Lentils: This should work with any type of lentils except Puy Lentils (French lentils, small dark brown/black ones because they hold their shape). Red, yellow, brown, green. The color of the soup will just be a bit different.

Cook times vary slightly as well so just start checking if the lentils are done at around 30 minutes.

I urge you to make this with dried lentils if you can. Better texture and flavor compared to canned. However, to make this with canned lentils, use 2 x 400g/14oz cans of lentils (drained and rinsed) and reduce the broth by 1 cup. Simmer the liquid for 20 minutes before adding the lentils then cook with lentils for another 15 minutes (don't want to cook canned lentils for too long otherwise they will turn into mush).

2. Storage: This freezes extremely well! Or keep it in the fridge for 3 to 5 days.

3. Nutrition per serving.

NUTRITION INFORMATION:

Serving:421g Calories:311cal (16%)
Carbohydrates:48g (16%) Protein:18g (36%)
Fat:5g (8%) Sodium:111mg (5%)
Potassium:925mg (26%) Fiber:22g (92%)
Sugar:5g (6%) Vitamin A:1930IU (39%) Vitamin

C:11.5mg (14%) Calcium:73mg (7%)
Iron:6mg (33%)

CHAPTER 4

PREPARING FOR SOLID FOODS

Signs your baby is ready for solid foods

Introducing your baby to solid foods, sometimes called complementary feeding or weaning, should start when your baby is around 6 months old.

In the beginning, how much your baby eats is less important than getting them used to the idea of eating.

They'll still be getting most of their energy and nutrients from breast milk or first infant formula.

Giving your baby a variety of foods, alongside breast or formula milk, from around 6 months of age will help set your child up for a lifetime of healthier eating.

Gradually, you'll be able to increase the amount and variety of food your baby eats until they can eat the same foods as the rest of the family, in smaller portions.

If your baby was born prematurely, ask your health visitor or GP for advice on when to start introducing solid foods.

Why wait until around 6 months to introduce solids?

It's a good idea to wait until around 6 months before introducing solid foods because:

- breast milk or first infant formula provides the energy and nutrients your baby needs until they're around 6 months old (except vitamin D in some cases)
- if you're breastfeeding, feeding only breast milk up to around 6 months of age will help protect your baby against illness and infections
- waiting until around 6 months gives your baby time to develop so they can cope fully with solid foods – this includes solid foods made into purées, cereals, and baby rice added to milk
- your baby will be more able to feed themselves

- your baby will be better at moving food around their mouth, chewing and swallowing it – this may mean they'll be able to progress to a range of tastes and textures (such as mashed, lumpy, and finger foods) more quickly, and may not need smooth, blended foods at all

Signs your baby is ready for solid foods

There are 3 clear signs which, when they appear together from around 6 months of age, show your baby is ready for their first solid foods alongside breast milk or first infant formula.

They'll be able to:

- stay in a sitting position and hold their head steady

- co-ordinate their eyes, hands, and mouth so they can look at the food, pick it up, and put it in their mouth by themselves

- swallow food (rather than spit it back out)

The following behaviors can be mistaken by parents as signs that their baby is ready for solid foods:

- chewing their fists

- waking up in the night (more than usual)

- wanting extra milk feeds

These are all normal behaviors for babies and not necessarily a sign that they're hungry or ready to start solid food.

Starting solid foods will not make your baby any more likely to sleep through the night. Sometimes a little extra milk will help until they're ready for solid foods.

How to start solid foods

In the beginning, your baby will only need a small amount of food before their usual milk feed.

Do not worry about how much they eat. The most important thing is getting them used to new tastes and textures, and learning how to move solid foods around their mouths and how to swallow them.

They'll still be getting most of their energy and nutrients from breast milk or infant formula.

There are some foods to avoid giving to your baby. For example, do not add sugar or salt (including stock cubes and gravy) to your baby's food or cooking water.

Babies should not eat salty foods as it's not good for their kidneys, and sugar can cause tooth decay.

Tips to get your baby off to a good start with solid foods:

- Eating is a whole new skill. Some babies learn to accept new foods and textures more quickly than others. Keep trying, and give your baby lots of encouragement and praise.

- Allow plenty of time, especially at first.

- Go at your baby's pace and let them show you when they're hungry or full. Stop when your baby shows signs that they've had enough. This could be firmly closing their mouth or turning their head away. If you're using a spoon, wait for your baby to open their mouth before you offer the food. Do not force your baby to eat. Wait until the next time if they're not interested this time.

- Be patient and keep offering a variety of foods, even the ones they do not seem to like. It may take 10 tries or more for your baby to get used to new foods, flavors, and textures. There will be days when they eat more, some when they eat less, and then days when they reject everything. Do not worry, this is perfectly normal.

- Let your baby enjoy touching and holding the food. Allow them to feed themselves, using their fingers, as soon as they show an interest. If you're using a spoon, your baby may like to hold it or another spoon to try feeding themselves.

- Keep distractions to a minimum during mealtimes and avoid sitting your baby in front of the television, phone, or tablet.

- Show them how you eat. Babies copy their parents and other children. Sit down together for family mealtimes as much as possible.

Texture progression

Once you've started introducing solid foods from around 6 months of age, try to move your baby on from puréed or blended foods to mashed, lumpy, or finger foods as soon as they can manage them.

This helps them learn how to chew, move solid food around their mouth and swallow.

Some babies like to start with mashed, lumpy, or finger foods.

Other babies need a little longer to get used to new textures, so may prefer smooth or blended foods on a spoon at first.

Just keep offering them lumpy textures and they'll eventually get used to it.

When introducing your baby to solid foods, it's important to take extra care to not put them at risk.

Key food safety and hygiene advice:

- always wash your hands before preparing food and keep surfaces clean
- cool hot food and test it before giving it to your baby
- wash and peel fruit and raw vegetables
- avoid hard foods like whole nuts, raw carrots, or apple
- remove hard pips and stones from fruits, and bones from meat or fish
- cut small, round foods, like grapes and cherry tomatoes, into small pieces
- eggs produced under the British Lion Code of Practice (stamped with the red lion) are considered very low risk for salmonella and safe for babies to eat partially cooked

Always stay with your baby when they're eating in case they start to choke.

Choking is different from gagging. Your baby may gag when you introduce solid foods.

This is because they're learning how to deal with solid foods and regulate the amount of food they can manage to chew and swallow at one time.

If your baby is gagging:

- their eyes may water
- they might push their tongue forward (or out of their mouth)
- they might retch to bring the food forward in their mouth or vomit

Equipment checklist

- High chair. Your baby needs to be sitting safely in an upright position (so they can swallow properly). Always use a securely fitted safety harness in a high chair. Never leave babies unattended on raised surfaces.
- Plastic or pelican bibs. It's going to be messy at first!

- Soft weaning spoons are gentler on your baby's gums.

- Small plastic bowl. You may find it useful to get a special weaning bowl with a suction base to keep the bowl in place.

- First cup. Introduce a cup from around 6 months and offer sips of water with meals. Using an open cup or a free-flow cup without a valve will help your baby learn to sip and is better for their teeth.

- A messy mat or newspaper sheets under the high chair to catch most of the mess.

- Plastic containers and ice cube trays can be helpful for batch cooking and freezing small portions.

Feeding your baby: from 0 to 6 months

Breast milk is the best food your baby can have during their first 6 months of life.

It's free, always available, and at the perfect temperature, and is tailor-made for your baby.

First infant formula is the only suitable alternative if you do not breastfeed or choose to supplement breast milk.

Other kinds of milk or milk substitutes, including cows' milk, should not be introduced as a main drink until 12 months of age.

"Follow-on" formula is not suitable for babies under 6 months, and you do not need to introduce it after 6 months.

Babies do not need baby rice to help them move to solid foods or sleep better.

When using a bottle, do not put anything (such as sugar or cereals) in it other than breast milk or infant formula.

Vitamins for babies

It's recommended that breastfed babies are given a daily supplement containing 8.5 to 10 micrograms (µg) of vitamin D from birth, whether or not you're taking a supplement containing vitamin D yourself.

Babies having 500mls (about a pint) or more of formula a day should not be given vitamin supplements.

This is because the formula is fortified with vitamin D and other nutrients.

All children aged 6 months to 5 years should be given vitamin supplements containing vitamins A, C, and D every day.

Feeding your baby: from around 6 months

When they first start having solid foods, babies do not need 3 meals a day. Babies have tiny tummies, so start by offering them small amounts of food (just a few pieces, or teaspoons of food).

Pick a time that suits you both, when you do not feel rushed and your baby is not too tired.

Start offering them food before their usual milk feed as they might not be interested if they're full, but do not wait until your baby is too hungry.

Allow plenty of time and let your baby go at their own pace.

Keep offering different foods, even foods your baby has already rejected.

It can take 10 tries or more before your baby will accept a new food or texture, particularly as they get older.

Your baby will still be getting most of their energy and nutrients from breast milk or first infant formula.

Breast milk or infant formula should be their main drink during the first year. Do not give them whole cows' (or goats' or sheep's) milk as a drink until they're 1 year old.

You can continue breastfeeding for as long as you both want.

Introduce a cup from around 6 months and offer sips of water with meals. Using an open cup or a free-flow cup without a valve will help your baby learn to sip and is better for their teeth.

First foods

You might want to start with single vegetables and fruits.

Try mashed or soft cooked sticks of parsnip, broccoli, potato, yam, sweet potato, carrot, apple or pear.

Include vegetables that are not sweet, such as broccoli, cauliflower, and spinach.

This will help your baby get used to a range of flavors (rather than just the sweeter ones, like carrots and sweet potato) and might help prevent them from being fussy eaters as they grow up.

Make sure any cooked food has cooled right down before offering it to your baby.

Foods containing allergens (such as peanuts, hens' eggs, gluten, and fish) can be introduced from around 6 months of age, 1 at a time, and in small amounts so you can spot any reaction.

Cows' milk can be used in cooking or mixed with food from around 6 months of age, but should not be given as a drink until your baby is 1 year old.

Full-fat dairy products, such as pasteurized cheese and plain yogurt or fromage frais, can be given from around 6 months of age. Choose products with no added sugar.

Remember, babies do not need salt or sugar added to their food (or cooking water).

Finger foods

As soon as your baby starts solid foods, encourage them to be involved in mealtimes and have fun touching, holding, and exploring food.

Let them feed themselves with their fingers when they want to. This helps develop fine motor skills and hand-eye coordination.

Your baby can show you how much they want to eat, and it gets them familiar with different types and textures of food.

Offering your baby finger foods at each meal is a good way to help them learn to self-feed.

Finger food is food that's cut up into pieces big enough for your baby to hold in their fist with a bit sticking out.

Pieces about the size of your finger work well.

Start with finger foods that break up easily in their mouth and are long enough for them to grip.

Avoid hard food, such as whole nuts or raw carrots and apples, to reduce the risk of choking.

Examples of finger foods include:

- soft cooked vegetables, such as carrot, broccoli, cauliflower, parsnip, butternut squash

- fruit (soft, or cooked without adding sugar), such as apple, pear, peach, melon, banana

- grabbable bits of avocado

- cooked starchy foods, such as potato, sweet potato, cassava, pasta, noodles, chapatti, rice

- pulses, such as beans and lentils

- fish without bones

- hardboiled eggs

- meat without bones, such as chicken and lamb

- sticks of pasteurized full-fat hard cheese (choose lower salt options)

Baby-led weaning

Baby-led weaning means giving your baby only finger foods and letting them feed themselves from the start instead of feeding them puréed or mashed food on a spoon.

Some parents prefer baby-led weaning to spoon-feeding, while others do a combination of both.

There's no right or wrong way. The most important thing is that your baby eats a wide variety of food and gets all the nutrients they need.

There's no more risk of choking when a baby feed themselves than when they're fed with a spoon.

Feeding your baby: from 7 to 9 months

From about 7 months, your baby will gradually move towards eating 3 meals a day (breakfast, lunch, and tea), in addition to their usual milk feeds, which may be around 4 a day (for example, on waking, after lunch, after tea and before bed).

As your baby eats more solid foods, they may want less milk at each feed or even drop a milk feed altogether.

If you're breastfeeding, your baby will adapt their feeds according to how much food they're having.

As a guide, formula-fed babies may need around 600ml of milk a day.

Gradually increase the amount and variety of food your baby is offered to ensure they get the energy and nutrients they need.

Try to include food that contains iron, such as meat, fish, fortified breakfast cereals, dark green vegetables, beans, and lentils, at each meal.

Your baby's diet should consist of a variety of the following:

- fruit and vegetables, including ones with bitter flavors, such as broccoli, cauliflower, spinach and cabbage

- potatoes, bread, rice, pasta, and other starchy foods

- beans, pulses, fish, eggs, meat, and other non-dairy sources of protein

- pasteurized full-fat dairy products, such as plain yogurt and cheese (choose lower salt options)

As your baby becomes a more confident eater, remember to offer them more mashed, lumpy, and finger foods.

Providing finger foods as part of each meal helps encourage infants to feed themselves, develop hand and eye coordination, and learn to bite off, chew, and swallow pieces of soft food.

Remember, babies do not need salt or sugar added to their food (or cooking water).

Feeding your baby: from 10 to 12 months

From about 10 months, your baby should now be having 3 meals a day (breakfast, lunch, and tea), in addition to their usual milk feeds.

Around this age, your baby may have about 3 milk feeds a day (for instance, after breakfast, after lunch, and before bed).

Breastfed babies will adapt their milk consumption as their food intake changes.

As a guide, babies fed infant formula will drink about 400ml daily.

Remember that formula-fed babies should take a vitamin D supplement if they're having less than 500ml of formula a day.

All breastfed babies should take a vitamin D supplement.

By now, your baby should be enjoying a wide range of tastes and textures.

They should be able to manage a wider range of finger foods and be able to pick up small pieces of food and move them to their mouth. They'll use a cup with more confidence.

Lunches and teas can include a main course, and a fruit or unsweetened dairy-based dessert, to move eating patterns closer to those of children over 1 year.

As your baby grows, eating together as a family encourages them to develop good eating habits.

Remember, babies do not need salt or sugar added to their food (or cooking water).

Feeding your baby: from 12 months
From 12 months, your child will be eating 3 meals a day containing a variety of different foods, including:

- a minimum of 4 servings a day of starchy food, such as potatoes, bread and rice

- a minimum of 4 servings a day of fruit and vegetables

- a minimum of 350ml milk or 2 servings of dairy products (or alternatives)

- a minimum of 1 serving a day of protein from animal sources (meat, fish, and eggs) or 2 from vegetable sources (dhal, beans, chickpeas and lentils)

Your child may also need 2 healthy snacks in between meals.

Go for things like:

- fresh fruits, such as apples, bananas, or small pieces of soft, ripe, peeled pear or peach

- cooked or raw vegetables, such as broccoli florets, carrot sticks or cucumber sticks

- pasteurized plain full-fat yogurt

- sticks of cheese (choose a lower salt option)

- toast, pitta, or chapatti fingers

- unsalted and unsweetened rice or corn cakes

The World Health Organization recommends that all babies be breastfed for up to 2 years or longer.

You can keep breastfeeding for as long as it suits you both, but your child will need less breast milk to make room for more food.

Once your child is 12 months old, infant formula is not needed and toddler milk, growing-up milk, and goodnight milk are also unnecessary.

Your baby can now drink whole cows' milk. Choose full-fat dairy products, as children under 2 years old need the vitamins and extra energy found in them.

From 2 years old, if they're a good eater and growing well, they can have semi-skimmed milk.

From 5 years old, 1% fat and skimmed milk is OK.

You can give your child unsweetened calcium-fortified milk alternatives, such as soya, oat, or almond drinks, from the age of 1 as part of a healthy, balanced diet.

Children under 5 years old should not be
given rice drinks because of the levels of arsenic
in these products.

CHAPTER 5

RECIPES FOR NEWBORNS (6-12 MONTHS)

Your infant discovers a whole new world when they begin to eat solid food. You're probably at a loss over what to give your kid, whether you're attempting baby-led weaning or the conventional spoon-feeding approach. Although preparing your baby's food can seem intimidating at first, it's quite simple and can even end up being less expensive than purchasing prepared foods.

These baby food recipes range from thin purees to complete finger foods for each phase of your solid feeding adventure.

Baby food recipes for 6 to 8 months

Around six months of age, babies are usually ready to start eating solid meals. Being able to sit up, controlling their head well, and displaying an interest in food are indicators that they are ready. An indication that your kid is ready is when they watch you eat, open their mouth when you give them a spoonful, or even try to take food from your plate.

Any pureed food with only one component can be given to your infant at first, such as bananas, berries, or many of the foods on this list.

The most common allergens—fish, wheat, eggs, soy, peanuts, tree nuts, sesame, and dairy—are the exceptions. It is advisable to start your infant off with low-allergy meals, such as pureed chicken or apples. You can begin introducing items that may cause allergies after you are certain they can tolerate those foods.

Serve a common allergy to your kid for three to five days before introducing a different kind of food. In this manner, it will be simpler to determine the reason for any adverse reaction your kid may have.

Try these baby food recipes for your 6- to 8-month-old:

- Apple and pear sauce

- Baby oats with prunes

- Butternut squash puree

- Green pea puree

- Mango and banana puree

- Peach or nectarine puree

- Roasted pears

- Sweet potato puree

- Turkey or chicken puree

- Whipped cauliflower

- Yogurt and berry swirl

- Zucchini puree

Baby food recipes for 9 to 12 months

By the time your baby is about 9 months old, they're ready for some more complex dishes — often, you'll find yourself feeding them whatever you and the rest of your family are eating.

While you're expanding your baby's eating horizons, remember they still don't have that many teeth and can't chew hard or crunchy produce like raw carrots — and be on the lookout for choking hazards, like whole grapes and popcorn. But there are still plenty of other options for babies at this age: flaky salmon, ground beef, roasted vegetables, baked potatoes, pasta dishes... the list goes on.

It's OK if the baby doesn't enjoy trying different textures. Offering your kid a variety of foods and persevering in your efforts are crucial at any age. Continue providing food to your baby even if they initially don't like it. It can take up to 20 attempts to get them to eat it.

At this age, your baby should also be ready to attempt finger foods, such as sliced bananas, toasted oat cereal in the shape of an O, or properly cooked spaghetti broken into bite-sized pieces that are about ¼ of an inch in size. Some of the recipes below, such as the whipped cauliflower, guacamole, and hummus, are great as finger food dips to help your baby begin to eat on their own. Naturally, it will be untidy, but it's a perfect opportunity for them to work on their hand-eye coordination and their newly acquired pincer grasp.

Try adding spices to your baby's food if you're game for some additional culinary explorations. Fresh herbs and other spices are acceptable (a little extra salt is permissible), even though it is not advised to give newborns added sugar or salt until they are at least two years old. Try putting some rosemary or cinnamon in their ground beef or oats.

Your kid might even like slightly spicy food if you want to try new flavors but steer clear of anything with a lot of added sugar, salt, or processing. (If you enjoy spicy cuisine and nursed your baby while doing so, your infant may even develop a natural tolerance to spice.)

Try these recipes for your 9- to 12-month-old:

- Asparagus risotto

- Baby guacamole

- Barley and mushroom mash

- Broccoli and cauliflower cheese

- Chicken curry with green beans and zucchini

- Coconut milk rice pudding with blueberry compote

- Homemade hummus

- Lentil and spinach stew

- Pasta with spinach and ricotta

- Oatmeal with apples

- Quinoa, black beans, and corn

- Rice with peas, carrots, and egg

- Root veggie mash

- Salmon, asparagus, and peas

- Shepherd's pie

- Smashed chickpea and butternut squash chili

- Tomato and avocado scramble

- Tropical fruit salad

Recipe 1: Pureed Carrots

Like sweet potato and winter squash, carrot puree makes a great stage 1 food for babies because it can easily be pureed until thin. Carrots are also low on the allergy scale and easily digested by a tiny tummy.

Carrot Nutrition for Young Children

How wholesome carrots are as a first meal! They are rich in beta-carotene, an antioxidant that appears red and orange and which the body metabolizes to vitamin A. It is well known that vitamin A strengthens the immune system and improves eye health. In addition, carrots provide fiber, iron, calcium, and vitamin C, all of which can support a baby's regular bowel motions.

Which Sort of Carrots to Cut

I prefer using whole, fresh carrots that are organic. To prepare and cook the carrots, simply give them a thorough wash and peel. Although peeling them is an additional step, I do advise doing so to get rid of any dirt or pesticide residue. I also believe that the carrots taste better after the peel is removed. When the peel is on, it tastes earthy to me. You can also use tiny carrots, which already have the peels removed, which speeds up the cutting process.

How to Make Carrot Puree

1. Peel and chop carrots.
2. Cook the carrot chunks by steaming, boiling, or roasting.
3. Transfer cooked carrots to a blender or food processor. I've been loving my Vita-mix for blending up baby food. It gets the purees super smooth!
4. Blend until smooth, adding breast milk, formula, or water to thin – the carrot puree will likely be a bit too thick for stage 1 eaters without adding some sort of liquid to thin the puree. I like using breast milk or formula for extra nutrients, but you can use water as well (water used for the steaming or boiling process works great).

5. Let carrot puree cool and serve right away or portion into storage containers or ice cube trays for later use.
6. Carrot puree can be stored in the fridge for 3 days or in the freezer for 3 months.

How to Store Carrot Baby Food

After the carrot puree has reached the desired consistency, allow it to cool before transferring it into ice cube trays or BPA-free storage containers. I've been utilizing these 4 oz glass storage containers and silicone ice cube trays. Because you may thaw one cube at a time, the ice cube trays are ideal for younger babies who aren't ingesting as much food. For larger babies who are taking more than one ounce at a time, however, the 4-ounce jars are excellent.

I recently purchased the WeeSprout glass storage containers designed especially for baby food, but we already have the ice cube trays. I like that the jars are made of glass rather than plastic, so there's no need to worry about BPA, and that they have measures printed on the side. They are safe to use in the microwave, freezer, and dishwasher. Additionally, they have vibrant lids that you can use to write the item and date using a dry-erase marker.

You can store the fresh carrot puree in the refrigerator for up to three days or freeze it for up to three months.

Remember to Label

Before keeping any baby food you prepare, I strongly advise labeling it! The speed at which you forget the day you prepared food after it's in the freezer or refrigerator is astounding.

How to Reheat or Thaw Frozen Carrot Puree

To thaw frozen pureed carrots, I recommend taking the jar out of the freezer the night before you want to use it so it can defrost in the fridge overnight. If you need to use it right away, you can thaw it using a water bath. Some people will recommend microwaving the frozen puree using the defrost seating but I prefer these two methods:

- Defrost in the refrigerator: Place frozen puree cubes into a jar or baby's serving dish, cover, and place in the refrigerator overnight. If you stored the puree in a jar or storage container, simply place the jar in the fridge.
- Water bath: Place frozen pureed cubes in a small container and set in another larger container with warm water. Replace the water as needed. Once defrosted, portion the food into individual bowls, cover, and refrigerate until serving.

Be sure to use any of the defrosted food within 48 hours of being defrosted and do not re-freeze.

Baby Food Combinations with Carrots

Once your baby is ready for stage 2 foods that are combinations, you can blend different fruits and veggies into the carrot puree. Here are some ideas of foods and spices that pair well with carrots.

- Green veggies – peas, broccoli, green beans, zucchini, spinach

- Orange veggies – butternut squash, sweet potatoes
- Fruits – apples, peaches, pears
- Carbs – brown rice, lentils, quinoa
- Protein – beef, chicken
- Herbs and Spices – cinnamon, ginger, cardamom, cumin, paprika, nutmeg, curry, mint

Recipe 2: Mashed Avocado and Banana

To make this Banana Avocado Baby Puree, you'll need the following ingredients:

Banana: although we recommend using a ripe banana for this Banana Avocado Baby Puree, a not-so-ripe one will also do as the blender will do its magic. It might take a little longer but the outcome should be the same. A ripe banana will have a sweeter taste because the starches have turned into sugars with the ripening process so that's also one of the reasons we recommend it.

Avocado: if you don't have a ripe avocado that you can easily scoop out from the skin with a spoon just place the whole avocado with the banana in a paper bag the day before. The banana and the paper bag should speed up the process.

BANANA AVOCADO BABY PUREE NUTRITIONAL BENEFITS

Bananas: they're a great source of carbs (starches or simple sugars, depending on the stage of ripeness) and a wonderful source of multiple vitamins and minerals. Mainly B vitamins, and the minerals potassium and copper.

Avocado: it's our go-to fruit when we want to add some healthy fats and calories to the puree. Since it mainly consists of fats the calorie content per gram is higher than with most other fruits. It's also a great source of fat-soluble vitamins such as the antioxidant vitamin E.

Banana Avocado Baby Puree

HOW TO MAKE BANANA AVOCADO BABY PUREE

Banana and Avocado are two of the rare fruits that don't require any cooking for a 6-month-old baby.

Peel the banana. Simple as that. No washing, rinsing, drying. Just peel that banana.

Cut the avocado. There are numerous ways to cut the avocado and scoop out the flesh and I've pretty much tried all of them. So I'd like to tell you what I found to be the easiest way. Take a knife and cut the avocado lengthwise all around. That grabs the top half with one hand and the bottom with the other and twists in opposite directions. Divide the halves and take out the seed. Now simply scoop the flesh from both halves with a spoon. If you have an avocado slicer like this one, just skip everything I told you above and use your slicer.

Blend. Now that you've prepared both of your ingredients, just throw them in the blender. You'd probably want to cut the banana into a few pieces or just divide it with your fingers to make it a bit easier for the blender. Blend until smooth. You can add a tablespoon of water to make it smoother but it will most likely not need it.

Certain blenders were created just for baby food but we have always used this blender for both our baby foods and every day for our (adult) smoothies.

Serving size is just for guidance, if your baby needs more or less food please follow their cue.

POSSIBLE BANANA-AVOCADO VARIATIONS

These two foods come together so well that they don't even have to be made as a puree.

Mashed. If you're over the puree stage or transitioning from purees to finger food then this recipe is perfect if you modify the "how-to" part. Instead of putting in the blender, you can simply mash the food together. You'd probably want your banana and avocado to be a little bit riper here so that it's easier to mash.

Banana Avocado Baby Puree

Lumps. If you're just a step away from finger food, you can also blend or mash one-half of the banana and avocado leave the rest in pieces and then join. That way your child will get used to new textures.

Finger food. Both the banana and avocado are great finger food. Cut the avocado into longer sticks after you've scooped the flesh, or into small cubes if your baby has mastered the pincer grips.

To avoid sticky bananas being hard to grab, cut the banana in half, then simply press your finger through the middle. You should be left with 3 banana sticks that are easier to grab.

Fridge Life? 3 days

Freezable? 3 months

INGREDIENTS

1 ripe avocado

1 large banana

INSTRUCTIONS:

Peel the banana

Cut the avocado lengthwise all around and twist the halves in opposite ways

Divide the 2 avocado halves and remove the seed

Scoop the avocado flesh from the skin of both halves with a spoon

Put both the banana and avocado flesh in a blender and blend until smooth

NUTRITION:

Calories: 107kcal

Carbohydrates: 11g

Protein: 1g

Fat: 7g

Saturated Fat: 1g

Polyunsaturated Fat: 1g

Monounsaturated Fat: 5g

Sodium: 4mg

Potassium: 349mg

Fiber: 4g

Sugar: 4g

Vitamin A: 92IU

Vitamin C: 8mg

Calcium: 8mg

Iron: 1mg

CONCLUSION

Two essential qualities that can have a big impact on our lives are consistency and patience.

Understanding that things don't happen all at once is the key to patience. It's about learning to move with life's natural flow, not against it, and accepting it. Being patient enables us to make sound judgments, maintain our composure under pressure, and remain composed in the face of hardship. Reminding us that wonderful things come slowly.

Contrarily, consistency is the resolve to carry out a regular action, regardless of its size, to accomplish a bigger objective. It involves creating routines, processes, and behaviors that support our long-term growth. Our daily activities towards our relationships, jobs, health, and personal development are all examples of consistency.

Patience and consistency together are a formidable combination. While consistency guarantees that we are making consistent development, patience serves as a reminder to maintain our composure.

Being a mother is a wonderful adventure that is full of intense love, hardships, and happy moments. Nutritious self- and baby-care is one of the most important parts of this trip.

Always keep in mind that caring for your health also means caring for your child. Maintaining a healthy diet, drinking plenty of water, and getting adequate sleep are not only self-care practices; they are also loving gestures toward your child.

Remember to treasure these times spent together when you feed your child. Every meal is a chance for you and your kid to grow closer, express your love, and support each other's physical development. It's a relationship more than it is diet.

If things don't always go as planned, that's acceptable. There may be days when the baby is cranky, you're exhausted, or you just need a break. It's alright. You're doing fantastically, and remember to treat yourself with kindness.

Savour every second, every smile, every tiny hold. These are the times when all the difficulties are worthwhile. You are feeding a life, not just a body, and that is cause for celebration.